Secret to an Everlasting Love:

Unlock the New Love Language to Win and Hold His Heart

Roselia J. Clark

Purpose of the Book

Welcome to "Secret to an Everlasting Love: Unlock the New Love Language to Win and Hold His Heart." This book is designed to help you discover and implement a revolutionary approach to love and communication in your relationship. By understanding and applying the new love language, you'll be able to deepen your connection, keep the spark alive, and build a lasting, fulfilling relationship with the man you love.

Overview of the New Love Language Concept

The concept of love languages, has transformed the way many people view relationships. While the original five love languages are incredibly valuable, this book introduces a new love language that addresses the evolving dynamics of modern relationships. This new love language encompasses elements of the traditional ones but also incorporates fresh, innovative approaches to understanding and expressing love.

Table of Contents

Chapter 10: Sustaining Love Through Lifelong Commitment

How to Use This Book

Each chapter of this book builds on the previous one, providing you with a comprehensive guide to mastering the new love language. You'll find practical tips, real-life examples, and actionable advice to help you apply these concepts to your relationship. Take your time to digest each chapter, practice the techniques, and observe how your relationship transforms.

Chapter 1: The Evolution of Love Languages

Traditional Love Languages vs. the New Love Language

Love languages, as popularized by Gary Chapman, traditionally include **acts of service**, **words of affirmation, quality time, physical touch, and receiving gifts.** These languages focus on how individuals express and receive love, shaping the dynamics of relationships for decades.

However, the landscape of relationships has evolved. The New Love Language takes a progressive approach by emphasizing not only how love is expressed but also how emotional needs are understood. It delves deeper into the nuances of emotional intelligence, mutual respect, and continuous growth within relationships.

Why the New Love Language Matters
Today: In today's fast-paced world, where
digital communication often replaces
face-to-face interactions, the New Love
Language offers a renewed perspective on
fostering meaningful connections. It
addresses the complexities of modern
relationships, where emotional intimacy and
mutual understanding are increasingly
valued.

By exploring the evolution of love languages
and introducing the concept of the New
Love Language, this chapter sets the stage
for readers to reconsider how they approach
communication and emotional connection
in their own relationships. It encourages a
shift towards a more holistic and adaptive
framework that aligns with contemporary
relationship dynamics.

Chapter 2: Emotional Intelligence and Relationship Dynamics

The Role of Emotional Intelligence in Relationships

Emotional intelligence (EI) forms the cornerstone of healthy relationship dynamics. This chapter explores how EI enables individuals to recognize, understand, and manage their own emotions, as well as those of their partners. By enhancing EI, couples can navigate conflicts more effectively, express empathy, and build deeper connections based on mutual emotional support.

Understanding Your Own Emotional Needs

Self-awareness is key to identifying core emotional needs such as validation, security, or intimacy and how these needs influence your behaviors and interactions within relationships.

Recognizing and Responding to Your
Partner's Emotional Needs

Effective relationships thrive on mutual
understanding and responsiveness to each
other's emotional needs. This section
provides practical strategies for recognizing
subtle cues and signals of emotional needs
in partners. By fostering empathy and active
listening, couples can create a supportive
environment where emotional intimacy
flourishes.

Chapter 3: Communication Strategies for Lasting Connection

Effective Communication: Beyond Words

Communication extends beyond verbal exchanges. This chapter explores non-verbal communication, including body language and tone of voice, which often convey more profound meanings than words alone. By mastering these subtleties, couples can enhance the clarity and depth of their communication.

Non-verbal cues such as facial expressions, gestures, and posture play a significant role in conveying emotions and intentions. Understanding and interpreting these cues accurately can prevent misunderstandings and foster empathy in relationships. Practical exercises are provided to help readers improve their non-verbal communication skills and deepen their connection with their partners.

Active Listening and Empathic Responding

Active listening involves fully concentrating, understanding, responding, and then remembering what is being said. Empathetic responding means expressing that understanding by giving appropriate feedback. This chapter emphasizes the importance of active listening in building trust and intimacy.

Readers are advised to learn techniques such as paraphrasing, summarizing, and asking open-ended questions to demonstrate their attentiveness and validate their partner's feelings. Through empathetic responding, couples create a supportive environment where emotions are acknowledged and shared openly, strengthening their bond.

Resolving Conflict Constructively

Conflict is inevitable in any relationship, but how it is managed determines its impact. This section explores constructive conflict resolution strategies that promote understanding and growth rather than escalation. Techniques such as "I-statements," collaborative problem-solving, and taking breaks during heated discussions are discussed in detail.

By approaching conflicts with empathy and a willingness to understand each other's perspectives, couples can navigate differences more effectively. Practical exercises and case studies illustrate successful conflict resolution techniques in action, empowering readers to apply these strategies in their relationships.

Chapter 4: Building Trust and Resilience

The Importance of Trust in Relationships

Trust forms the foundation of every healthy and enduring relationship. This chapter explores the multifaceted nature of trust, encompassing reliability, transparency, and emotional vulnerability. Readers gain insights into how trust is built over time through consistent actions, open communication, and mutual respect.

Trust allows couples to feel secure and confident in their partnership, fostering intimacy and commitment. Practical tips are provided for cultivating trust, such as setting clear boundaries, honoring promises, and being accountable for one's actions. Case studies highlight the transformative power of trust in overcoming challenges and deepening connection.

Strategies for Building and Maintaining Trust

Building trust requires ongoing effort and commitment from both partners. This section outlines proactive strategies for cultivating trust in relationships, including honest communication, demonstrating reliability, and showing empathy during difficult times.

Readers learn how to address breaches of trust sensitively and effectively, rebuilding confidence and restoring harmony in their relationships. By fostering a culture of trust and forgiveness, couples create a resilient foundation that withstands adversity and strengthens their bond over time.

Navigating Challenges and Strengthening Resilience

Challenges and setbacks are inevitable in every relationship. This chapter explores resilience as the ability to adapt, bounce back from adversity, and grow stronger together. Readers discover resilience-building techniques such as cultivating optimism, practicing self-care, and seeking support from each other and trusted individuals.

By embracing challenges as opportunities for personal and relational growth, couples deepen their resilience and fortify their commitment to each other. Real-life examples illustrate how couples have overcome obstacles, demonstrating the transformative potential of resilience in sustaining lasting love.

Chapter 5: Love and Self-Discovery

Embracing Self-Discovery within Your Relationship

In every relationship, personal growth and self-discovery are vital for both partners to thrive individually and together. This chapter explores how couples can support each other's journey of self-discovery while nurturing a strong, connected partnership.

Self-discovery within a relationship involves understanding one's own desires, goals, and values, and how these align with the partnership. It encourages individuals to explore their identities and aspirations while fostering an environment of mutual support and encouragement.

Each person in a relationship brings unique dreams and aspirations. Couples need to create space for these aspirations to flourish, whether they relate to career ambitions, personal interests, or personal growth. By supporting each other's journeys, partners can cultivate a sense of fulfillment and satisfaction that enriches their relationship.

Navigating Differences and Growth Together:

Self-discovery often involves navigating differences between partners and embracing growth opportunities. It requires open communication, empathy, and a willingness to support each other through changes and challenges. By embracing each other's evolving identities, couples can deepen their connection and build a resilient foundation for their relationship.

Embracing self-discovery within a relationship is a journey of mutual growth and understanding. It encourages partners to celebrate each other's individuality.

Chapter 6: Practical Applications and Exercises

Reflections on Your Relationship Journey

Self-reflection and introspection are powerful tools for strengthening relationships. This chapter encourages couples to reflect on their journey together, celebrating milestones and learning from challenges to deepen their connection and appreciation for each other.

Reflecting on the relationship journey allows couples to acknowledge the progress they've made, understand their shared experiences, and recognize areas for growth. It fosters gratitude and strengthens emotional bonds by creating a shared narrative of love and resilience.

Creating a Timeline of Significant Moments: Creating a timeline of significant moments in the relationship helps couples revisit important milestones, from the first date to major life events. It prompts discussions about cherished memories, challenges overcome, and future aspirations, fostering a deeper appreciation for the journey they've taken together.

Sharing Gratitude and Acknowledgment: Expressing gratitude for each other's contributions and strengths cultivates positivity and appreciation within the relationship. Couples can take turns sharing specific qualities they admire in each other and how these qualities have enriched their lives.
Reflections on the relationship journey serve as a reminder of the love, resilience, and growth that have shaped the partnership. It reinforces commitment and encourages couples to continue nurturing their bond through shared experiences and mutual understanding.

Chapter 7: Real-Life Examples and Case Studies

Case Studies of Successful Relationships

Real-life examples provide inspiration and practical insights into how couples navigate challenges, cultivate resilience, and sustain meaningful connections over time. This chapter presents case studies of couples who have overcome adversity and strengthened their relationships through dedication, communication, and mutual support.

Case studies offer a glimpse into the lives of real couples who have faced and triumphed over challenges in their relationships. They demonstrate the principles and practices discussed throughout the book in action, showcasing the transformative power of love and commitment.

Case Study 1: Overcoming Communication Barriers:
This case study explores how a couple struggled with communication issues early in their relationship but learned to listen actively, express vulnerability, and prioritize understanding. Through couples counseling and dedicated effort, they rebuilt trust and established healthier communication patterns that strengthened their bond.

Case Study 2: Navigating Life Transitions Together:
In this case study, a couple shares their journey of supporting each other through significant life changes, such as career shifts, relocation, or health challenges. By prioritizing empathy, flexibility, and shared decision-making, they navigated transitions with resilience and deepened their commitment to each other.

Learning from Challenges and Transformations:
Each case study concludes with key lessons learned and actionable insights for readers to apply in their relationships. It highlights the importance of perseverance, mutual respect, and continuous growth in sustaining a loving and enduring partnership.

Real-life examples and case studies demonstrate that every relationship encounters obstacles, but with dedication, communication, and mutual support, couples can overcome challenges and emerge stronger than before. I encourage others to apply these lessons in their relationships, fostering resilience, understanding, and lasting love.

Chapter 8: The Author's PerspectiveInsights from a Relationship Counselor

Drawing from my expertise as a relationship counselor, this chapter offers valuable insights and wisdom gained from years of experience working with couples. It provides practical advice and strategies for maintaining a healthy, fulfilling relationship based on understanding, empathy, and effective communication.

My professional journey in the field of relationship counseling so far, I will tell you that the importance of continuous learning and adapting strategies to meet the evolving needs of couples cannot be overemphasized

Principles of Successful Relationships:
Key principles for building and sustaining successful relationships are; trust, communication, empathy, and mutual respect. These principles form the

foundation for navigating challenges and fostering intimacy in long-term partnerships.

The author's perspective underscores the importance of seeking professional guidance when needed and emphasizes that successful relationships are built on continuous effort, mutual growth, and a commitment to nurturing love and understanding.

Chapter 9: The Power of Shared Values and Goals

Aligning Values and Goals in Relationships

Shared values and goals form the bedrock of a strong, enduring relationship. This chapter explores how couples can identify and align their core values, aspirations, and life goals to create a unified vision for their future together.

Shared values are fundamental beliefs and principles that guide individuals in their decisions and behaviors. When couples share similar values, they are better equipped to navigate challenges and make decisions that align with their mutual aspirations.

Identifying Core Values:
Identifying your core values and that of your partner is very essential because the core

values shape your perspectives on relationships, family, career, and personal growth. Understanding each other's values promotes empathy and strengthens the foundation of trust and respect within the relationship.

For example: A couple discussing their future together and realize they have differing views on financial planning and career priorities, what should they do?

It's not far-fetched; They should engage in open and honest conversations to understand each other's perspectives and underlying values. Through compromise and mutual respect, they develop a shared approach to financial management and career goals that honors both of their aspirations. I hope that's clear

Setting Mutual Goals:
Setting mutual goals allows couples to create a roadmap for their relationship and

individual growth. Whether they focus on career advancement, family planning, travel, or personal development, shared goals provide a sense of purpose and unity in working towards a common vision.

Chapter 10: Sustaining Love Through Lifelong Commitment

Nurturing Long-Term Love and Commitment

Building a lasting and fulfilling relationship requires ongoing effort, dedication, and a shared commitment to growth and understanding. This final chapter explores strategies for nurturing love, fostering resilience, and sustaining a deep emotional connection throughout the journey of lifelong commitment.

Lifelong commitment is about more than just staying together; it's about continuously investing in each other's happiness, growth, and well-being. This chapter examines the principles and practices that contribute to the longevity and vibrancy of relationships.

Cultivating Emotional Intimacy:

Emotional intimacy forms the cornerstone of a strong, enduring relationship. Couples learn to cultivate emotional intimacy through open communication, vulnerability, and mutual trust. They share their innermost thoughts, fears, and aspirations, creating a safe space for authentic connection and understanding.

Renewing Romance and Passion: Maintaining romance and passion is essential for keeping the spark alive in long-term relationships. Couples explore ways to prioritize romance, whether through date nights, surprise gestures, or shared adventures. They continue to nurture physical affection and intimacy, keeping their relationship vibrant and fulfilling.

Navigating Challenges and Adversities: Every relationship faces challenges, from external stressors to internal conflicts. Couples learn strategies for navigating challenges together, including effective communication, problem-solving skills, and resilience-building techniques. They embrace challenges as opportunities for growth and learning, supporting each other through difficult times.

Celebrating Milestones and Achievements: Celebrating milestones, both big and small, reinforces appreciation and gratitude within the relationship. Couples reflect on their journey together, acknowledging achievements and milestones such as anniversaries, career successes, or personal milestones. They express pride and admiration for each other's accomplishments, fostering a sense of shared pride and joy.

Sustaining love through lifelong commitment requires dedication, communication, and a willingness to grow together. By nurturing emotional intimacy, renewing romance, navigating challenges, and celebrating achievements, couples create a foundation of love and resilience that enriches their lives and deepens their connection over time. This chapter encourages couples to embrace the journey of lifelong commitment with optimism, resilience, and a shared sense of purpose, ensuring a love that lasts a lifetime.

www.ingramcontent.com/pod-product-compliance
Lightning Source LLC
Chambersburg PA
CBHW051724250726
48653CB00008B/3189